Understanding Youth Suicide: A Comprehensive Guide for Healthcare Workers

Copyright Page

TITLE: Understanding Youth Suicide: A Comprehensive Guide for Healthcare Workers

1ST Edition

ISBN: 9798223082347

Table of Contents

Understanding Youth Suicide: A Comprehensive Guide for Healthcare Workers

By Roberto Miguel Rodriguez

Chapter 1: Introduction

Overview of Youth Suicide

Youth suicide is a critical issue that demands the attention of healthcare workers across various niches in the United States. This subchapter aims to provide a comprehensive understanding of youth suicide, focusing on its prevalence and various factors contributing to it. By delving into specific niches such as LGBTQ+ youth, bullying-related suicide, minority youth, rural youth, Native American youth, foster care system, college students, cyberbullying, mental health disparities, and military family youth, we can gain a deeper insight into the multifaceted nature of this problem.

The United States continues to face alarming rates of youth suicide, making it imperative for healthcare workers to be well-informed and equipped to address this crisis. Understanding the prevalence of youth suicide is the first step towards effective intervention and prevention strategies. By analyzing the latest data and statistics, healthcare workers can identify trends and patterns that shed light on the most at-risk populations.

One such group is LGBTQ+ youth, who face unique challenges and higher rates of suicide compared to their heterosexual peers. This section explores the various stressors and discrimination that contribute to the increased vulnerability of LGBTQ+ youth and offers strategies for providing culturally competent care and support.

Bullying-related youth suicide is another pressing concern. Healthcare workers need to grasp the detrimental effects of bullying on mental health and how it can lead to suicidal ideation and behaviors. By understanding the dynamics of bullying and implementing preventative measures, healthcare workers can help create safer environments for vulnerable youth.

Additionally, minority youth, rural youth, Native American youth, and those in the foster care system are disproportionately affected by suicidal tendencies. This subchapter delves into the unique challenges these populations face, such as limited access to mental healthcare and higher rates of trauma, and provides strategies for culturally sensitive interventions.

Furthermore, college students, who often experience intense academic pressure and transitions, are susceptible to mental health struggles and suicidal ideation. Healthcare workers in educational settings should be aware of the resources available to support these students and recognize the signs of distress.

In the digital age, cyberbullying has emerged as a significant contributor to youth suicide. By examining the impact of online harassment and providing guidelines for prevention and intervention, healthcare workers can assist in safeguarding young individuals from the harmful effects of cyberbullying.

Mental health disparities, particularly among marginalized communities, are closely linked to youth suicide rates. Healthcare workers must be attuned to these disparities and advocate for equitable access to mental health services for all youth.

Lastly, the unique challenges faced by military families, including frequent relocations, deployment-related stress, and loss, contribute to increased suicide rates among their youth. Healthcare workers must be knowledgeable about the support systems available to military families and provide comprehensive mental health care to mitigate these risks.

By delving into these niches of youth suicide, healthcare workers can gain a deeper understanding of the complex factors contributing to this crisis and develop effective strategies for prevention and intervention. It is crucial to approach this issue with compassion, cultural sensitivity, and a commitment to fostering resilience in young individuals.

Importance of Understanding Youth Suicide

In today's society, youth suicide has become an alarming issue that demands the attention of healthcare workers. Understanding the complexities and factors that contribute to youth suicide is essential for healthcare professionals who play a vital role in preventing and addressing this crisis. This subchapter will delve into the significance of comprehending youth suicide, focusing on various niches within the United States, including LGBTQ+ youth, bullying-related cases, minorities, rural areas, Native American communities, foster care system, college students, cyberbullying, mental health disparities, and military families.

Youth suicide in the United States has reached disturbing levels, making it crucial for healthcare workers to have a comprehensive understanding of this phenomenon. By gaining insights into the specific challenges faced by different groups, healthcare professionals can develop targeted prevention strategies and provide effective support systems. For instance, LGBTQ+ youth face unique stressors and are at a higher risk of suicide due to discrimination, social rejection, and internalized stigma. Healthcare workers must be equipped with the knowledge and skills to create safe and inclusive environments for these individuals.

Bullying-related youth suicide is another pressing issue that healthcare workers need to address. Understanding the link between bullying and suicide can help identify warning signs and implement preventive measures. Similarly, healthcare professionals must recognize the unique mental health challenges faced by minority youth, Native American communities, and those living in rural areas. By acknowledging their unique circumstances and providing culturally sensitive care, healthcare workers can reduce the risk of suicide in these populations.

The foster care system also presents a vulnerable group at a higher risk of suicide. Healthcare workers need to understand the various stressors faced by children in foster care and provide appropriate mental health support. Additionally, college students, who often face academic pressure and increased stress levels, require specialized interventions to prevent suicide.

In the digital age, cyberbullying has emerged as a significant concern. Healthcare workers must familiarize themselves with the impact of online harassment on youth mental health and develop strategies to address this issue effectively. Furthermore, mental health disparities and the impact of military family dynamics on youth suicide cannot be overlooked. Healthcare workers must be aware of these disparities and provide accessible and tailored mental health services to those in need.

By understanding the specific contexts and challenges faced by different groups, healthcare workers can play a crucial role in preventing youth suicide. This subchapter will equip healthcare professionals with the necessary knowledge to recognize risk factors, implement preventive measures, and provide appropriate support to those at risk. Through comprehensive understanding and targeted interventions, we can work together to reduce youth suicide rates and create a safer environment for our young population.

Role of Healthcare Workers in Youth Suicide Prevention

Introduction:

Youth suicide is a pressing issue that affects various marginalized populations in the United States. As healthcare workers, we have a crucial role to play in preventing youth suicide and promoting mental well-being among vulnerable groups such as LGBTQ+ youth, minorities, rural communities, Native Americans, foster care system, college students, victims of cyberbullying, individuals facing mental health disparities, and military families. This subchapter explores the specific roles healthcare workers can undertake to address the unique challenges faced by these populations.

1. Creating Safe Spaces:

Healthcare workers must establish safe and supportive environments where young individuals can discuss their mental health concerns without fear of judgment or discrimination. By fostering open communication, we can encourage them to seek help when needed. This is especially important for LGBTQ+ youth, as they may face additional stressors related to their sexual orientation or gender identity.

2. Identifying Warning Signs:

Healthcare workers should be trained to recognize the warning signs of suicidal ideation in youth. Through comprehensive assessments and screenings, we can identify those at risk and provide appropriate interventions. Special attention should be given to minority youth, who may face unique challenges such as racial discrimination or cultural stigma surrounding mental health.

3. Collaboration and Referrals:

Collaboration with other professionals, such as mental health specialists, social workers, and educators, is vital in addressing the complex factors contributing to youth suicide. Healthcare workers must ensure seamless referrals to appropriate resources and services, such as counseling, support groups, or helplines, to meet the diverse needs of at-risk populations.

4. Education and Prevention Programs:

Healthcare workers should actively engage in educating youth, families, and communities about suicide prevention strategies. This includes raising awareness about the impact of bullying, cyberbullying, and mental health disparities. By organizing workshops, training sessions, and community outreach programs, we can equip individuals with the necessary skills to recognize and respond to suicidal behaviors.

5. Policy Advocacy:

Healthcare workers have a responsibility to advocate for policy changes that address the underlying factors contributing to youth suicide. This may involve advocating for anti-bullying measures in schools, improving access to mental health services in underserved areas, or promoting cultural competence training within the foster care system.

Conclusion:

As healthcare workers, our role in youth suicide prevention is multifaceted and demands a compassionate and comprehensive approach. By creating safe spaces, identifying warning signs, collaborating with other professionals, conducting education and prevention programs, and advocating for policy changes, we can make a significant impact in reducing youth suicide rates among marginalized populations. Together, let us work towards creating a society where every young person feels valued, supported, and equipped with the tools to overcome life's challenges.

Chapter 2: Understanding Youth Suicide in the United States

Statistics and Trends

In order to effectively address the issue of youth suicide, healthcare workers must have a comprehensive understanding of the statistics and trends surrounding this devastating phenomenon. By examining the data and trends related to youth suicide in various populations, we can develop targeted interventions and support systems to prevent further loss of young lives. This subchapter will explore key statistics and trends in several niche areas of youth suicide in the United States, including LGBTQ+ youth, bullying-related suicides, minority youth, rural youth, Native American youth, youth in the foster care system, college students, victims of cyberbullying, individuals affected by mental health disparities, and youth from military families.

The statistics surrounding youth suicide in the United States are alarming. According to recent data, suicide is the second leading cause of death among young people aged 10 to 24. LGBTQ+ youth face a significantly higher risk, with studies showing that they are almost five times more likely to attempt suicide compared to their heterosexual peers. Bullying also plays a pivotal role in youth suicide, with victims being at a higher risk of suicidal ideation and attempts. Minority youth, particularly African American and Hispanic youth, are disproportionately affected by suicide, and cultural factors must be taken into account when developing prevention strategies.

Rural youth face unique challenges, including limited access to mental healthcare resources, social isolation, and economic disadvantage, which contribute to higher suicide rates. Native American youth also experience alarmingly high rates of suicide, with cultural loss, historical trauma, and limited healthcare resources playing significant roles. The foster care system presents another concerning aspect, as youth in foster care are at an increased risk of suicide due to adverse childhood experiences and instability.

College students, despite being in a seemingly supportive environment, face numerous stressors that can lead to mental health issues and suicide. The rise of technology has also brought new challenges, with cyberbullying contributing to the risk of suicide among young people. Mental health disparities among different populations, including low-income individuals and those with limited access to healthcare, exacerbate the risk of suicide. Lastly, youth from military families often face unique stressors, such as parental deployment and frequent relocations, which can increase the risk of suicide.

By understanding these statistics and trends, healthcare workers can work towards developing targeted prevention strategies, improving access to mental healthcare resources, and providing culturally sensitive support systems to address the specific needs of these vulnerable populations. Together, we can strive to reduce the incidence of youth suicide and ensure that no young life is lost to this preventable tragedy.

Risk Factors and Warning Signs

Understanding the risk factors and warning signs associated with youth suicide is crucial for healthcare workers in order to effectively identify and intervene in potentially life-threatening situations. This subchapter aims to provide healthcare workers with comprehensive knowledge and insights into the various risk factors and warning signs that are prevalent in different populations of youth in the United States.

In the context of youth suicide in the United States, it is important to recognize the unique challenges faced by LGBTQ+ youth. Research consistently shows that LGBTQ+ youth are at a higher risk of suicidal ideation and attempts due to factors such as discrimination, stigma, and social isolation. Healthcare workers must be aware of the specific warning signs in this population, including expressions of hopelessness, withdrawal, and a sudden decline in academic performance.

Bullying-related youth suicide is another critical area that healthcare workers need to understand. Bullying can have severe consequences on the mental health of young individuals, leading to increased risk of suicide. Recognizing signs of bullying, such as social withdrawal, changes in behavior, and frequent absenteeism, is pivotal in preventing tragic outcomes.

Minority youth, particularly those from marginalized communities, are also more susceptible to suicidal ideation and attempts. Understanding the cultural and social factors that contribute to this vulnerability is essential for healthcare workers. Warning signs may include changes in sleep patterns, sudden weight loss or gain, and expressions of feeling trapped or hopeless.

Rural areas face unique challenges in addressing youth suicide, with limited access to mental health resources and higher rates of substance abuse. Healthcare workers in these regions must be trained to identify signs of depression, isolation, and substance misuse, as these are common risk factors in rural youth.

Native American youth experience disproportionately high rates of suicide compared to other ethnic groups. Healthcare workers must be aware of the historical trauma, substance abuse, and limited access to mental health services that contribute to this crisis. Warning signs may include engagement in risky behaviors, increased substance use, and a sudden loss of interest in cultural activities.

Further topics covered in this subchapter include the foster care system and youth suicide, college student suicide, cyberbullying and youth suicide, mental health disparities, and military family youth suicide. By familiarizing healthcare workers with the unique risk factors and warning signs associated with these niches, this subchapter aims to equip them with the necessary knowledge and skills to intervene effectively and save lives.

In conclusion, understanding the risk factors and warning signs associated with youth suicide is crucial for healthcare workers. By recognizing the specific challenges faced by different populations, healthcare workers can play a vital role in preventing tragic outcomes and promoting mental wellness in vulnerable youth across the United States.

Protective Factors and Resilience

In the face of the alarming rise in youth suicide rates across various demographics in the United States, it is crucial for healthcare workers to understand the concept of protective factors and resilience. By identifying and strengthening these factors, we can better support and empower vulnerable youth populations, such as LGBTQ+ individuals, minority groups, college students, Native Americans, and those in the foster care system.

Protective factors encompass a range of internal and external factors that enhance an individual's resilience and reduce their vulnerability to suicidal thoughts and behaviors. These factors can be seen as a shield that buffers against the risk factors associated with youth suicide. While risk factors may include mental health disorders, bullying, social isolation, and family instability, protective factors offer a counterbalance and promote psychological well-being.

One crucial protective factor is the presence of a strong support network. Healthcare workers can play a pivotal role in fostering connections between youth and their families, friends, teachers, and mentors. By strengthening these relationships, we can provide a safety net for vulnerable individuals, ensuring they have someone to turn to during times of crisis.

Additionally, mental health support and access to quality healthcare services are vital protective factors. By increasing awareness and reducing the stigma surrounding mental health, healthcare workers can facilitate early intervention and ensure that at-risk youth receive the care they need. Moreover, providing culturally competent and inclusive mental health services is essential, as it addresses the unique challenges faced by minority groups and LGBTQ+ individuals.

Building resilience is another key aspect of preventing youth suicide. Resilience refers to an individual's ability to bounce back from adversity and navigate life's challenges. Healthcare workers can promote resilience by fostering coping skills, problem-solving abilities, and emotional regulation techniques in young individuals. By equipping them with these tools, we empower them to face difficulties head-on and develop a sense of purpose and self-worth.

Furthermore, community engagement and prevention programs are crucial in promoting protective factors and resilience. Healthcare workers can collaborate with schools, community organizations, and policymakers to implement evidence-based prevention strategies that address specific risk factors prevalent in their respective regions. By addressing issues such as cyberbullying, mental health disparities, and the unique challenges faced by rural and Native American communities, we can create a comprehensive approach to youth suicide prevention.

In conclusion, protective factors and resilience are vital components in combating the alarming rates of youth suicide in the United States. By fostering strong support networks, providing accessible mental health services, promoting resilience, and engaging communities, healthcare workers can make a significant impact in preventing youth suicide across various demographics. Together, we can create a safer and more supportive environment for the youth, ensuring their well-being and fostering a brighter future.

Impact of Youth Suicide on Communities

Youth suicide is a pressing public health issue that has far-reaching consequences on various communities in the United States. The impact of these tragic losses is felt not only by the families and friends of the victims but also by healthcare workers and the broader community. Understanding the profound effects of youth suicide on communities is crucial for healthcare workers to develop effective prevention and intervention strategies. This subchapter explores the different facets of this impact on various niches, including LGBTQ+ youth, bullying-related suicide, minority youth, rural communities, Native American communities, foster care system, college students, cyberbullying, mental health disparities, and military families.

One significant impact of youth suicide on communities is the emotional toll experienced by those left behind. Families and friends are devastated by the loss of a loved one, struggling with grief, guilt, and unanswered questions. Healthcare workers play a crucial role in providing support and counseling to these individuals, helping them navigate the complex emotions and facilitating their healing process.

In the LGBTQ+ community, youth suicide rates are alarmingly high due to the unique challenges faced by these individuals. Discrimination, bullying, and lack of acceptance contribute to feelings of isolation and hopelessness. Healthcare workers must be sensitive to the specific needs of LGBTQ+ youth, offering inclusive and nonjudgmental support to prevent further tragedies.

Bullying-related suicide is another disturbing issue affecting communities nationwide. The relentless torment and humiliation experienced by victims of bullying can lead to severe psychological distress and suicidal ideation. Healthcare workers can collaborate with schools and organizations to implement anti-bullying campaigns and provide mental health resources to support affected youth.

Minority youth, particularly in marginalized communities, face additional stressors that contribute to their vulnerability to suicide. Socioeconomic disparities, limited access to mental healthcare, and cultural stigma surrounding mental health further compound the challenges these youth face. Healthcare workers must address these disparities by advocating for equal access to mental health services and culturally competent care.

Rural communities often lack sufficient mental health resources, making it difficult for youth to access timely and appropriate support. The isolation and limited opportunities in these areas can exacerbate feelings of hopelessness. Healthcare workers can bridge this gap by promoting telehealth services and collaborating with local organizations to provide mental health outreach programs.

Native American communities experience disproportionately high rates of youth suicide, rooted in historical trauma, cultural disconnection, and limited resources. Healthcare workers need to engage with these communities respectfully, acknowledging their unique cultural and historical contexts, and working collaboratively to develop prevention strategies.

The foster care system presents additional risk factors for youth suicide, including instability, trauma, and difficulties in forming stable relationships. Healthcare workers should advocate for improved support services within the foster care system, including mental health resources and trauma-informed care.

On college campuses, the pressure to succeed academically, social isolation, and the transition to adulthood can contribute to an increased risk of suicide among students. Healthcare workers can collaborate with universities to implement comprehensive mental health programs, increasing awareness, and providing accessible support services.

Cyberbullying is another growing concern, with the pervasiveness of technology enabling harassment and humiliation to continue beyond the confines of school. Healthcare workers must educate both youth and parents about the potential dangers of cyberbullying and provide strategies for prevention and intervention.

Mental health disparities in underserved communities contribute to higher rates of suicide among youth. Healthcare workers should advocate for equitable access to mental health services and work to reduce the stigma surrounding mental health concerns.

Finally, military families face unique challenges, including frequent relocations, deployment-related stress, and the impact of trauma. Healthcare workers can collaborate with military support organizations to provide targeted mental health services and support systems for military youth.

In conclusion, the impact of youth suicide on communities is vast and varied. Healthcare workers must be equipped with a comprehensive understanding of the specific challenges faced by different niches to effectively address this issue. By working collaboratively with communities, implementing prevention strategies, and providing accessible support services, healthcare workers can make a significant difference in reducing youth suicide rates and supporting affected communities.

Chapter 3: LGBTQ+ Youth Suicide in the United States

Unique Challenges Faced by LGBTQ+ Youth

The struggles faced by LGBTQ+ youth are particularly unique and deserve special attention in the context of youth suicide. Healthcare workers must have a comprehensive understanding of these challenges in order to effectively support and advocate for this vulnerable population.

One of the primary challenges LGBTQ+ youth face is the pervasive discrimination and stigma they encounter on a daily basis. This can lead to feelings of isolation, rejection, and shame, which significantly contribute to their risk for suicide. Many LGBTQ+ youth are subjected to bullying, both in person and online, which further exacerbates their distress. Studies have shown that LGBTQ+ youth are at a higher risk for bullying-related suicide compared to their heterosexual counterparts.

Moreover, LGBTQ+ youth often face rejection from their families, which can have devastating consequences. Family support is crucial for the well-being of young individuals, and the absence of it puts LGBTQ+ youth at a significantly increased risk for suicide. Additionally, religious and cultural beliefs may further compound the challenges faced by these individuals, as they may not find acceptance or understanding within their communities.

Access to appropriate healthcare is another significant challenge for LGBTQ+ youth. Many face barriers to accessing mental health services due to financial constraints, lack of insurance coverage, or healthcare providers who are not knowledgeable or supportive of their unique needs. This lack of access to affirming care can further contribute to their feelings of hopelessness and increase their risk for suicide.

Furthermore, LGBTQ+ youth in rural areas or those from minority communities face additional challenges. These individuals often lack access to LGBTQ+-affirming resources and support systems, which further exacerbates their feelings of isolation and distress. Native American LGBTQ+ youth, for example, experience disproportionately high rates of suicide due to the intersection of cultural factors, historical trauma, and discrimination.

To effectively address the unique challenges faced by LGBTQ+ youth, healthcare workers must undergo specialized training that focuses on LGBTQ+ cultural competency and provide affirming and supportive care. It is crucial to create safe spaces within healthcare settings where LGBTQ+ youth can openly discuss their experiences and receive appropriate mental health support.

By recognizing and addressing the unique challenges faced by LGBTQ+ youth, healthcare workers can play a vital role in preventing youth suicide within this vulnerable population. It is imperative that healthcare systems and providers work towards creating inclusive and affirming environments that prioritize the mental health and well-being of LGBTQ+ youth.

Contributing Factors to LGBTQ+ Youth Suicide

LGBTQ+ youth face unique challenges and are at a higher risk of suicide compared to their heterosexual peers. Understanding the contributing factors to LGBTQ+ youth suicide is crucial for healthcare workers to provide effective support and interventions. This subchapter explores the various factors that contribute to LGBTQ+ youth suicide in the United States and provides insight into these specific niches: Youth Suicide in the United States, LGBTQ+ Youth Suicide in the United States, Bullying-Related Youth Suicide in the United States, Minority Youth Suicide in the United States, Rural Youth Suicide in the United States, Native American Youth Suicide in the United States, Foster Care System and Youth Suicide in the United States, College Student Suicide in the United States, Cyberbullying and Youth Suicide in the United States, Mental Health Disparities and Youth Suicide in the United States, and Military Family Youth Suicide in the United States.

One of the primary contributing factors to LGBTQ+ youth suicide is the pervasive discrimination and stigma they face. LGBTQ+ youth often experience rejection, bullying, and harassment, both in their schools and communities, which can lead to feelings of isolation, depression, and hopelessness. This discrimination can be particularly severe for minority LGBTQ+ youth, who face the challenge of intersecting identities and multiple forms of discrimination based on race, ethnicity, and sexual orientation.

Bullying is another significant factor contributing to LGBTQ+ youth suicide. Research consistently shows that LGBTQ+ youth are at a higher risk of being bullied compared to their heterosexual peers. The relentless bullying and victimization can have devastating effects on their mental health and overall well-being. Moreover, cyberbullying, facilitated by social media platforms, exacerbates the harm caused by traditional forms of bullying, leading to increased feelings of despair and self-harm.

The mental health disparities faced by LGBTQ+ youth are also contributing factors to their increased risk of suicide. Many LGBTQ+ youth struggle with internalized homophobia, shame, and fear due to societal attitudes and expectations. These negative emotions, coupled with limited access to affirming mental health services, create significant barriers to seeking help and support.

Additionally, the foster care system and college environments can pose unique challenges for LGBTQ+ youth. Those in foster care may face discrimination and a lack of supportive resources, increasing their vulnerability to suicide. Similarly, college students may experience a hostile campus climate, lack of inclusive policies, and limited access to

LGBTQ+ support services, making them more susceptible to mental health issues and suicide.

Awareness of these contributing factors is essential for healthcare workers to provide appropriate care and support to LGBTQ+ youth. By addressing discrimination, promoting inclusive environments, and providing culturally competent mental health services, healthcare workers can play a crucial role in reducing LGBTQ+ youth suicide rates in the United States.

Supportive Strategies for LGBTQ+ Youth

Introduction:

The rates of youth suicide in the United States are alarming, especially among certain marginalized populations such as LGBTQ+ youth. Healthcare workers play a crucial role in supporting and advocating for these vulnerable individuals. This subchapter aims to provide healthcare workers with supportive strategies specifically tailored to address the unique challenges faced by LGBTQ+ youth. By implementing these strategies, healthcare workers can contribute to reducing suicide rates among this population.

Creating a Safe and Inclusive Environment:

1. Educate Yourself: Healthcare workers should familiarize themselves with LGBTQ+ terminology, identities, and issues. This knowledge will help them better understand and connect with LGBTQ+ youth.

2. Use Inclusive Language: Ensure that your language is inclusive and avoids assumptions about gender or sexual orientation. Respect and affirm the gender identities and pronouns expressed by LGBTQ+ youth.

3. Establish Trust: Build a foundation of trust by actively listening to LGBTQ+ youth, validating their experiences, and creating a

non-judgmental environment. Make it clear that you are a supportive ally.

Enhancing Mental Health Support:

1. Provide Culturally Competent Care: Understand the unique mental health challenges faced by LGBTQ+ youth, including minority youth within this population. Tailor treatment plans to address their specific needs, such as exploring gender identity or dealing with discrimination.

2. Offer LGBTQ+ Affirmative Therapy: Connect LGBTQ+ youth with therapists who are knowledgeable and supportive of their identities. Affirmative therapy can help them navigate the challenges they face and build resilience.

3. Encourage Peer Support: Facilitate support groups or connect LGBTQ+ youth to local LGBTQ+ organizations. Peer support can provide a sense of belonging and reduce feelings of isolation.

Promoting Safety and Well-being:

1. Address Bullying: Advocate for anti-bullying policies in schools and educate staff on LGBTQ+ sensitivity training. Encourage LGBTQ+ youth to report bullying incidents and provide resources for self-defense.

2. Supportive Families: Work with families to create an accepting and supportive environment at home. Provide resources, information, and counseling to help families understand and accept their LGBTQ+ children.

3. Collaborate with Community Organizations: Partner with LGBTQ+ organizations and community centers to provide comprehensive support services. These organizations often offer resources, counseling, and safe spaces for LGBTQ+ youth.

Conclusion:

Healthcare workers have a crucial role in supporting LGBTQ+ youth and reducing suicide rates within this population. By creating safe and inclusive environments, enhancing mental health support, and promoting safety and well-being, healthcare workers can empower LGBTQ+ youth to lead fulfilling lives. Collaboration with community organizations and ongoing education will further strengthen their ability to provide effective and compassionate care.

Chapter 4: Bullying-Related Youth Suicide in the United States

Types and Effects of Bullying

Introduction:

Bullying is a pervasive issue that affects youth across various demographics in the United States. Its detrimental effects can lead to severe consequences, including an increased risk of youth suicide. As healthcare workers, it is imperative to understand the different types of bullying and their specific effects on various populations.

1. Types of Bullying:

a. Physical Bullying: This involves physical aggression such as hitting, pushing, or damaging personal belongings. Physical bullying can result in physical injuries and long-term psychological trauma.

b. Verbal Bullying: This type of bullying includes name-calling, teasing, or spreading rumors. Verbal bullying can cause emotional distress, low self-esteem, and feelings of isolation.

c. Relational Bullying: Also known as social bullying, this form involves manipulating relationships, ostracizing, or excluding individuals from social activities. Relational bullying can lead to social isolation, depression, and anxiety.

d. Cyberbullying: With the rise of technology, bullying has extended to the online realm. Cyberbullying involves sending hurtful messages, spreading rumors, or sharing embarrassing content through digital platforms. It can have devastating effects on mental health, including increased risk of suicide.

2. Effects of Bullying:

a. Psychological Effects: Bullying can cause a range of psychological issues such as depression, anxiety, post-traumatic stress disorder (PTSD), and suicidal ideation. Victims may experience feelings of hopelessness, helplessness, and overwhelming stress.

b. Academic Consequences: Bullying often leads to poor academic performance due to increased absenteeism, difficulty concentrating, and reduced motivation. It can hinder educational development and opportunities for success.

c. Social Effects: Victims of bullying may struggle to form healthy relationships, feel socially isolated, and experience difficulties in developing trust and emotional connections.

d. Long-term Impact: The effects of bullying can extend into adulthood, leading to chronic mental health issues, substance abuse, and a higher risk of self-harm or suicide.

Conclusion:

Understanding the types and effects of bullying is crucial for healthcare workers who aim to address the underlying factors contributing to youth suicide in the United States. By recognizing the signs and providing appropriate support, healthcare professionals can play a vital role in preventing the devastating consequences of bullying on the mental health and well-being of vulnerable populations, including LGBTQ+ youth, minority groups, those in the foster care system, college students, military families, and Native American communities. Additionally, addressing the impact of cyberbullying and mental health disparities is essential in creating a safer environment for all youth, ultimately reducing the risk of youth suicide in the United States.

Link between Bullying and Youth Suicide

Bullying has long been recognized as a significant risk factor for youth suicide. It is a complex issue that affects various populations, including LGBTQ+ youth, minority youth, rural youth, Native American youth, college students, and those in the foster care system. In recent years, cyberbullying has emerged as a particularly concerning form of bullying that can have devastating consequences. Healthcare workers play a vital role in understanding and addressing the link between bullying and youth suicide to prevent tragic outcomes.

Research consistently shows a strong association between bullying and suicidal ideation, attempts, and completed suicides among young people. Victims of bullying often experience high levels of emotional distress, depression, anxiety, and social isolation. These factors, combined with the inability to escape the torment, can lead to feelings of hopelessness and despair. It is crucial for healthcare workers to recognize the signs of bullying and intervene early to provide support and resources to vulnerable youth.

LGBTQ+ youth face unique challenges, as they are more likely to experience bullying and discrimination based on their sexual orientation or gender identity. The rates of suicide among LGBTQ+ youth are alarmingly high, emphasizing the urgent need for targeted interventions and inclusive healthcare practices. Healthcare workers must create safe and affirming spaces where LGBTQ+ youth can seek help without fear of judgment or stigma.

Similarly, minority youth, especially those from racial and ethnic minority groups, are disproportionately affected by bullying and its detrimental consequences. Cultural factors, prejudice, and discrimination contribute to the increased vulnerability of these individuals. Healthcare workers must be aware of these disparities and advocate for culturally sensitive approaches to suicide prevention and mental health support.

Rural youth, Native American youth, college students, and those in the foster care system face specific challenges that can exacerbate the link between bullying and suicide. The isolation, limited access to resources, and unique stressors experienced by these populations demand tailored interventions. Healthcare workers must collaborate with community organizations, educational institutions, and social services to develop comprehensive strategies that address the root causes of bullying and provide effective support systems.

Furthermore, the advent of technology and social media has given rise to cyberbullying, a pervasive form of harassment that can follow young people into their homes and personal lives. Healthcare workers must be knowledgeable about the impact of cyberbullying on mental health and educate both youth and parents on safe internet practices and coping strategies.

In conclusion, understanding the link between bullying and youth suicide is crucial for healthcare workers. By recognizing the specific challenges faced by different populations, healthcare workers can implement targeted interventions to prevent bullying and provide support to those at risk. Through collaboration, education, and advocacy, healthcare workers can play a pivotal role in reducing the devastating impact of bullying on young people's lives.

Prevention and Intervention Approaches for Bullying

Bullying is a pervasive issue affecting youth across various demographics in the United States. It has been identified as a significant risk factor for youth suicide, particularly among vulnerable populations such as LGBTQ+ youth, minority youth, rural youth, Native American youth, those in the foster care system, college students, youth affected by cyberbullying, and those from military families. Healthcare workers play a crucial role in understanding and addressing this problem to prevent youth suicide.

Prevention strategies for bullying should encompass a multi-faceted approach, involving collaboration between healthcare workers, educators, parents, and community members. Education and awareness programs need to be implemented in schools, colleges, and healthcare settings to foster a safe and inclusive environment. These programs should focus on promoting empathy, respectful communication, and conflict resolution skills among youth.

Early identification and intervention are vital in addressing bullying behaviors. Healthcare workers should be trained to recognize signs of bullying and engage in open conversations with youth who may be affected. It is essential to provide a supportive and non-judgmental environment, ensuring confidentiality and privacy. Screening tools can be utilized to assess the extent of bullying and its impact on mental health.

Intervention approaches should involve a comprehensive support system for victims, bullies, and bystanders. Victims of bullying may require counseling and mental health services to address the trauma they have experienced. Empowerment programs can help victims develop resilience and coping strategies. Bullies need interventions that focus on addressing the underlying issues contributing to their behavior, such as family dynamics or mental health problems. Bystanders should be encouraged to report incidents and be equipped with skills to safely intervene.

In cases of cyberbullying, healthcare workers should collaborate with technology experts to develop effective prevention and intervention strategies. This may involve promoting responsible online behavior, educating youth about the potential consequences of cyberbullying, and establishing reporting mechanisms for online abuse.

Furthermore, healthcare workers should advocate for policy changes at local, state, and national levels to address the root causes of bullying.

This could include implementing anti-bullying legislation, strengthening disciplinary measures, and promoting social inclusion initiatives.

In conclusion, prevention and intervention approaches for bullying require a comprehensive and collaborative effort from healthcare workers, educators, parents, and communities. By fostering a safe and inclusive environment, early identification, and targeted interventions, we can effectively reduce the risk of youth suicide associated with bullying.

Chapter 5: Minority Youth Suicide in the United States

Disparities and Vulnerabilities Faced by Minority Youth

In addressing the issue of youth suicide, it is crucial for healthcare workers to understand the disparities and vulnerabilities faced by minority youth in the United States. While suicide affects individuals across different demographics, certain groups face unique challenges that contribute to their increased risk.

One such group is LGBTQ+ youth, who are disproportionately affected by suicide compared to their heterosexual peers. LGBTQ+ youth often face bullying, rejection, and discrimination, which can lead to feelings of isolation and worthlessness. Healthcare workers must be aware of the specific needs of this population and provide inclusive and affirming care to support their mental well-being.

Another vulnerable group is minority youth, including African American, Hispanic, and Asian American communities. These communities often encounter systemic barriers such as poverty, limited access to healthcare, and cultural stigma surrounding mental health. These factors can exacerbate feelings of hopelessness and increase the risk of suicide. Healthcare workers must be sensitive to the cultural nuances and tailor their interventions to effectively address the unique challenges faced by minority youth.

Rural youth also face distinctive vulnerabilities. Living in remote areas often means limited access to mental health services and resources. Additionally, rural communities may have higher rates of substance abuse and limited social support networks, further adding to the risk of suicide. Healthcare workers must work collaboratively with community leaders and organizations to develop innovative approaches for reaching rural youth and providing them with the necessary support.

Native American youth also experience alarmingly high rates of suicide. Historical trauma, cultural disconnection, and limited resources contribute to their vulnerability. Healthcare workers need to engage with tribal communities, build trust, and develop culturally appropriate interventions that address the root causes of distress.

Youth in the foster care system and college students are two other groups at increased risk of suicide. These individuals often face significant transitions, loss, and trauma, which can further exacerbate existing mental health issues. Healthcare workers must be proactive in identifying and supporting these vulnerable populations, ensuring access to mental health services and providing a supportive environment.

Other key areas of concern include the impact of cyberbullying on youth suicide, mental health disparities among different racial and ethnic groups, and the challenges faced by youth in military families. Healthcare workers need to stay informed about these issues, engage in ongoing education, and collaborate with multidisciplinary teams to develop comprehensive strategies for prevention and intervention.

By understanding the disparities and vulnerabilities faced by minority youth, healthcare workers can better serve these populations and implement effective preventive measures. It is crucial to adopt a holistic approach that addresses the underlying social, cultural, and systemic factors contributing to youth suicide. By working together and advocating for change, healthcare workers can make a significant impact in reducing suicide rates among minority youth in the United States.

Cultural and Societal Factors Influencing Minority Youth Suicide

In recent years, the issue of youth suicide has become a pressing concern in the United States. It is a complex problem that affects various segments of the population, including minority youth. Understanding the cultural and societal factors that contribute to this phenomenon is crucial for healthcare workers who aim to prevent and address youth suicide effectively.

One significant factor influencing minority youth suicide is the experience of discrimination and prejudice. Minority youth often face systemic racism and social exclusion, which can have a profound impact on their mental health. The constant battle against discrimination can lead to feelings of hopelessness, despair, and a lack of belongingness, increasing their vulnerability to suicide.

Cultural norms and expectations also play a role in minority youth suicide. In some cultures, mental health issues are stigmatized, and seeking help for emotional distress is seen as a sign of weakness. This can prevent minority youth from reaching out for support, exacerbating their feelings of isolation and despair.

Additionally, the intersectionality of identities further compounds the risk for minority youth. For example, LGBTQ+ minority youth face unique challenges that can increase their susceptibility to suicide. The struggle to reconcile their sexual orientation or gender identity with societal expectations, along with the heightened rates of bullying and rejection, significantly contribute to their heightened risk.

Another influential factor is the lack of access to culturally competent mental healthcare. Minority youth often face barriers such as language barriers, limited healthcare resources in their communities, and a lack of awareness about available services. This hinders their ability to receive appropriate and timely mental health support, leaving them at a higher risk for suicide.

Addressing these cultural and societal factors requires a comprehensive approach. Healthcare workers must advocate for policies and programs that promote inclusivity, diversity, and equality. Culturally sensitive mental health services should be made available and accessible to minority youth, ensuring that their unique needs are met.

Education and awareness campaigns targeted towards minority communities can help reduce the stigma surrounding mental health and suicide. By promoting open dialogue and destigmatizing mental health issues, healthcare workers can encourage help-seeking behaviors and foster a supportive environment for minority youth.

In conclusion, cultural and societal factors significantly influence minority youth suicide rates in the United States. Healthcare workers must be aware of these factors to provide effective support and intervention. By addressing discrimination, stigma, and access barriers, we can work towards reducing the alarming rates of minority youth suicide and creating a more inclusive and supportive society for all.

Culturally Competent Interventions for Minority Youth

In addressing the complex issue of youth suicide, it is crucial for healthcare workers to recognize the unique challenges faced by minority youth in the United States. Culturally competent interventions play a pivotal role in providing effective support and prevention strategies tailored to the specific needs of these marginalized populations.

Minority youth are disproportionately affected by mental health disparities and are at a higher risk of suicide compared to their non-minority counterparts. Factors such as discrimination, acculturation stress, and the experience of multiple intersecting identities can contribute to their vulnerability. Therefore, healthcare workers must be equipped with the knowledge and skills to engage with these diverse communities in a culturally sensitive manner.

First and foremost, understanding the cultural context is essential for providing effective interventions. Healthcare workers should familiarize themselves with the cultural beliefs, values, and traditions of the minority communities they serve. This knowledge will enable them to establish trust, build rapport, and develop interventions that align with the cultural norms and preferences of these youth.

Additionally, healthcare workers should adopt a holistic approach that recognizes the intersectionality of a young person's identity. Minority youth often face multiple forms of discrimination based on their race, ethnicity, gender, sexual orientation, or socioeconomic status. By acknowledging and addressing these intersecting identities, healthcare workers can provide more comprehensive support and intervention strategies.

Community engagement and collaboration are crucial for implementing culturally competent interventions. Healthcare workers should actively involve community leaders, organizations, and stakeholders in the planning and implementation of suicide prevention programs. This collaborative approach ensures that interventions are culturally relevant, inclusive, and community-driven.

Moreover, healthcare workers must be mindful of the potential barriers faced by minority youth in accessing mental health services. Language barriers, lack of insurance, and limited culturally competent resources may hinder their ability to seek help. It is imperative for healthcare workers to address these barriers by providing language interpretation services, advocating for accessible and affordable mental health services, and actively seeking out community resources.

In conclusion, culturally competent interventions are essential for addressing the alarming rates of youth suicide among minority populations in the United States. Healthcare workers must strive to understand the cultural context, adopt a holistic approach, engage with the community, and address barriers to access. By doing so, they can provide effective and tailored support to help prevent youth suicide and promote mental well-being among minority youth.

Chapter 6: Rural Youth Suicide in the United States

Challenges and Risk Factors in Rural Communities

In recent years, youth suicide has become a pressing issue in the United States, affecting various segments of the population. While the causes of youth suicide are multifaceted, it is crucial to understand the unique challenges and risk factors faced by different communities. In this subchapter, we will explore the challenges and risk factors specifically associated with rural communities.

Rural communities often face distinct challenges that contribute to higher rates of youth suicide. One of the main challenges is limited access to mental healthcare services. Unlike urban areas, rural communities often lack sufficient mental health resources, including mental health professionals and treatment facilities. This scarcity of services can result in delayed or inadequate treatment for at-risk youth, exacerbating their vulnerability to suicide.

Another significant risk factor in rural communities is social isolation. Rural areas typically have smaller populations and limited social networks, making it more difficult for young people to find support and connection. The lack of peer support and social opportunities can increase feelings of loneliness and despair, leading to a higher risk of suicide.

Additionally, economic hardships prevalent in many rural communities can contribute to youth suicide. High poverty rates, limited job opportunities, and financial instability place significant stress on families and individuals. This economic strain can impact young people's mental health, increasing their vulnerability to suicidal thoughts and behaviors.

Moreover, substance abuse is a prevalent issue in rural areas, which further compounds the risk of youth suicide. Drug and alcohol misuse can lead to mental health problems and impulsive behaviors, both of which are associated with an increased risk of suicide. Limited access to substance abuse treatment and prevention programs in rural communities can exacerbate this issue.

Furthermore, cultural and societal factors unique to rural communities can also contribute to youth suicide. Stigma surrounding mental health, lack of awareness about available resources, and traditional gender roles that discourage help-seeking behaviors are all factors that may impede youth from seeking help or support.

Addressing the challenges and risk factors in rural communities requires a comprehensive and tailored approach. Healthcare workers must collaborate with community leaders, schools, and families to develop strategies that increase access to mental healthcare services, promote social connectedness, and address the economic and substance abuse issues prevalent in these areas.

By understanding and addressing the specific challenges faced by rural communities, healthcare workers can play a crucial role in preventing youth suicide and promoting the well-being of young people in these underserved areas.

Access to Mental Health Services in Rural Areas

Rural areas in the United States face unique challenges when it comes to accessing mental health services, and this is particularly concerning in the context of youth suicide. Healthcare workers play a crucial role in understanding and addressing these challenges to ensure that young people in rural communities receive the support they need. This subchapter explores the barriers faced by rural areas and provides strategies for improving access to mental health services.

One significant barrier to accessing mental health services in rural areas is the shortage of mental health professionals. Compared to urban areas, rural communities have a limited number of healthcare providers, leaving them underserved and at a disadvantage when it comes to mental health care. Healthcare workers need to be aware of this shortage and advocate for increased funding and incentives to attract mental health professionals to rural areas.

Transportation is another major obstacle in rural areas. Many young people in these communities may lack reliable transportation or live far away from mental health providers. Healthcare workers can address this issue by collaborating with local organizations and schools to establish transportation services specifically for mental health appointments. Telehealth and telepsychiatry can also be effective solutions, allowing young people to access mental health services remotely.

Stigma surrounding mental health is a pervasive problem in rural communities. Lack of awareness and understanding often leads to underutilization of mental health services. Healthcare workers must work to reduce stigma by providing education and community outreach programs. Building trust with families and community members is essential in breaking down barriers and encouraging help-seeking behaviors.

Another aspect to consider is the cultural and linguistic diversity in rural areas. Minority youth, including Native American youth, may face additional challenges due to cultural differences and a lack of culturally competent mental health services. Healthcare workers should strive to understand the unique needs and perspectives of these populations and work towards providing culturally sensitive care.

Finally, healthcare workers should collaborate with schools, community organizations, and local government to develop comprehensive mental health initiatives in rural areas. By establishing partnerships and integrating mental health services into existing systems, access to care can be improved and the overall well-being of young people in rural communities can be enhanced.

In conclusion, addressing the barriers to accessing mental health services in rural areas is crucial in preventing youth suicide. Healthcare workers have a vital role to play in advocating for increased resources, implementing innovative solutions, reducing stigma, and fostering community partnerships. By working together, we can ensure that young people in rural areas have access to the support they need to thrive.

Community-Based Approaches for Rural Youth Suicide Prevention

Rural communities in the United States face unique challenges when it comes to addressing youth suicide. Limited access to mental health resources, isolation, and stigma surrounding mental health issues are just a few factors that contribute to the higher rates of suicide among rural youth. To combat this crisis, community-based approaches have emerged as effective strategies for prevention and intervention.

One key aspect of community-based approaches is the involvement of various stakeholders, including healthcare workers, educators, parents, and community leaders. By working together, these individuals can create a comprehensive support network that addresses the specific needs of rural youth. This collaborative effort can help identify at-risk individuals, provide necessary resources, and promote mental health awareness within the community.

A crucial component of community-based approaches is the establishment of mental health programs and services within rural areas. This includes ensuring that mental health professionals are available and accessible to the youth population. Telehealth services, for example, can bridge the gap between rural communities and mental health providers, enabling youth to access support from the comfort of their homes.

Additionally, training programs can be implemented to educate healthcare workers and educators on identifying warning signs of suicide and providing appropriate interventions.

Another effective strategy is the incorporation of peer support programs. Peer support has proven to be highly beneficial for rural youth, as it provides a sense of belonging and understanding. By connecting young individuals who have experienced similar struggles, peer support programs offer a safe space where they can share their experiences and seek guidance from their peers. These programs can be facilitated through schools, community centers, or online platforms, ensuring accessibility for all rural youth.

Furthermore, community-based approaches should prioritize destigmatizing mental health issues. By fostering open conversations and promoting mental health literacy, rural communities can create an environment where seeking help is encouraged and accepted. This can be achieved through awareness campaigns, educational workshops, and community events that focus on mental health.

In conclusion, community-based approaches are critical for addressing the alarming rates of youth suicide in rural areas. By involving various stakeholders, establishing mental health programs, incorporating peer support, and destigmatizing mental health issues, healthcare workers and other individuals can make a significant impact on suicide prevention among rural youth. Through these collaborative efforts, we can create a supportive and resilient community that prioritizes the mental well-being of its young population.

Chapter 7: Native American Youth Suicide in the United States

Historical Context and Cultural Factors

Understanding the historical context and cultural factors surrounding youth suicide is crucial for healthcare workers to effectively address and prevent this growing public health concern. By examining these factors, healthcare professionals can gain a deeper understanding of the unique challenges faced by different populations, such as LGBTQ+ youth, minority youth, Native American youth, college students, and military families. This subchapter aims to provide a comprehensive overview of the historical and cultural factors influencing youth suicide in the United States across these diverse populations.

Historical Context:

To comprehend the current landscape of youth suicide, it is essential to explore the historical factors that have contributed to its prevalence. Historical events such as economic recessions, wars, and societal shifts have had a significant impact on mental health and suicide rates among young individuals. By understanding the historical context, healthcare workers can identify patterns and potential risk factors associated with youth suicide.

Cultural Factors:

Cultural factors play a pivotal role in shaping attitudes towards mental health, help-seeking behaviors, and social support networks. This subchapter will delve into the cultural factors that influence youth suicide, including the stigmatization of mental health issues, traditional gender roles, cultural norms surrounding sexuality, and the impact of social media. By recognizing and addressing these cultural aspects, healthcare professionals can tailor interventions and support systems that are sensitive to the needs of different cultural groups.

Specific Populations:

This subchapter will also provide insights into the unique challenges faced by specific populations, including LGBTQ+ youth, minority youth, Native American youth, college students, and military families. Each of these populations has distinct cultural, historical, and social factors that contribute to their increased vulnerability to youth suicide. By examining these factors, healthcare workers can develop targeted prevention strategies and interventions that address the specific needs of these populations.

Overall, understanding the historical context and cultural factors surrounding youth suicide is essential for healthcare workers to provide effective care and prevention strategies. By recognizing the unique challenges faced by different populations, healthcare professionals can work towards reducing youth suicide rates and promoting mental well-being among vulnerable groups.

Addressing the Unique Needs of Native American Youth

In recent years, there has been a growing concern over the rising rates of youth suicide in the United States, particularly among vulnerable populations such as LGBTQ+ youth, minority youth, and those living in rural areas. Among these at-risk groups, Native American youth stand out as one of the most affected. Understanding and addressing the unique needs of Native American youth is crucial in combatting the alarming rates of youth suicide within this community.

Native American youth suicide in the United States is a complex issue with deep-rooted historical, cultural, and socioeconomic factors. It is essential for healthcare workers to recognize and respect the cultural diversity within Native American communities. Engaging with tribal leaders, elders, and community members is crucial in gaining a comprehensive understanding of the challenges faced by Native American youth.

One of the key factors contributing to the high rates of youth suicide among Native Americans is the ongoing intergenerational trauma caused by historical events such as forced assimilation, colonization, and the displacement of Native American communities. This trauma often manifests in mental health issues, substance abuse, and feelings of hopelessness among Native American youth. Healthcare workers must be sensitive to this historical context and provide appropriate support and counseling services.

Another critical aspect of addressing the unique needs of Native American youth is ensuring access to culturally appropriate mental health care. Many Native American communities have limited resources and face geographical barriers to accessing healthcare services. Healthcare workers need to collaborate with tribal health organizations and establish culturally competent programs that integrate traditional healing practices and Western medicine.

Education plays a vital role in preventing youth suicide among Native Americans. Healthcare workers should actively engage with schools and community organizations to provide mental health awareness programs, suicide prevention training, and support systems. It is crucial to involve parents, teachers, and community leaders in these initiatives to create a holistic approach to addressing the mental health needs of Native American youth.

To effectively address the unique needs of Native American youth, healthcare workers must also advocate for policy changes at the federal, state, and tribal levels. These policies should focus on increasing funding for mental health services, improving access to healthcare facilities, and addressing the social determinants of health that contribute to the high rates of youth suicide in Native American communities.

In conclusion, addressing the unique needs of Native American youth is a pressing issue in combating the alarming rates of youth suicide in the United States. Healthcare workers play a crucial role in understanding the historical, cultural, and socioeconomic factors that contribute to these challenges. By engaging with tribal communities, providing culturally appropriate care, promoting mental health education, and advocating for policy changes, healthcare workers can make a significant impact in reducing youth suicide rates among Native American youth.

Collaborative Efforts with Native American Communities

In addressing the issue of youth suicide, it is crucial for healthcare workers to recognize the unique challenges faced by different communities. One such community that requires special attention is the Native American population in the United States. Native American youth suicide rates are alarmingly high, highlighting the urgent need for collaborative efforts to prevent and address this crisis effectively.

Historical trauma, cultural disconnection, poverty, and limited access to mental health resources are among the factors contributing to the high suicide rates among Native American youth. To address this issue, healthcare workers must engage in collaborative efforts with Native American communities to develop culturally sensitive and community-specific prevention strategies.

Firstly, it is essential for healthcare workers to establish strong relationships with tribal leaders, community members, and organizations. By actively listening and respecting the cultural values and practices of Native American communities, healthcare workers can build trust and gain valuable insights into the unique challenges faced by Native American youth. This collaboration will help in tailoring prevention and intervention programs to meet the specific needs of these communities.

Secondly, healthcare workers should work closely with Native American schools and educational institutions. By implementing suicide prevention programs within these settings, healthcare workers can reach a significant number of Native American youth. These programs should incorporate culturally relevant elements such as traditional healing practices, storytelling, and involvement of elders to promote resilience and mental well-being.

Thirdly, healthcare workers should advocate for increased funding and resources for mental health services in Native American communities. This can include supporting the establishment of mental health clinics within tribal lands, training more Native American mental health professionals, and providing culturally competent care to Native American youth.

Lastly, healthcare workers must engage in ongoing research and evaluation to assess the effectiveness of prevention efforts and identify areas for improvement. By collaborating with Native American communities and involving them in research initiatives, healthcare workers can ensure that the voices and experiences of Native American youth are represented in the development of evidence-based strategies.

In conclusion, addressing the high rates of youth suicide among Native American populations requires collaborative efforts between healthcare workers and Native American communities. By recognizing the unique challenges faced by these communities, engaging in culturally sensitive prevention strategies, advocating for increased resources, and conducting ongoing research, healthcare workers can make a substantial difference in reducing youth suicide rates among Native American youth.

Chapter 8: Foster Care System and Youth Suicide in the United States

Vulnerabilities and Trauma Experienced by Foster Youth

Introduction:

The foster care system plays a critical role in protecting and supporting vulnerable children and teens. However, it is essential for healthcare workers to understand the unique challenges faced by foster youth, as they are at a significantly higher risk of experiencing trauma and engaging in self-harming behaviors, including suicide. This subchapter aims to shed light on the vulnerabilities and trauma experienced by foster youth in the United States, providing healthcare workers with the knowledge and tools necessary to effectively address their needs.

Understanding the Challenges:

Foster youth often face a myriad of emotional, psychological, and social challenges that contribute to their increased vulnerability. Many have experienced abuse, neglect, or family disruption, leading to feelings of loss, abandonment, and a lack of stability. These early traumatic experiences can have long-lasting effects on their mental health and well-being.

Risk Factors for Foster Youth Suicide:

Numerous risk factors contribute to the higher rates of suicide among foster youth. These include a higher prevalence of mental health disorders such as depression, anxiety, and post-traumatic stress disorder (PTSD). The lack of consistent and nurturing relationships, frequent placement changes, and a sense of isolation further exacerbate their vulnerability. Additionally, the stigma associated with being in foster care often leads to feelings of shame and self-blame, compounding their emotional distress.

Addressing the Needs of Foster Youth:

Healthcare workers play a crucial role in identifying and addressing the unique needs of foster youth. This includes providing trauma-informed care, recognizing the signs of mental health issues, and facilitating access to appropriate mental health support services. Collaborating with social workers, therapists, and educators is vital in developing comprehensive care plans that address the specific challenges faced by foster youth.

Promoting Resilience and Protective Factors:

While foster youth face significant vulnerabilities, it is essential to highlight the protective factors that can mitigate their risk of suicide. Strong and supportive relationships with caring adults, access to appropriate mental health services, and stability in their living situations can greatly enhance their resilience. Healthcare workers can contribute to these protective factors by advocating for stable placements, providing ongoing emotional support, and empowering foster youth to build healthy coping strategies.

Conclusion:

Understanding the vulnerabilities and trauma experienced by foster youth is crucial for healthcare workers in effectively addressing their unique needs. By providing trauma-informed care, recognizing risk factors, and promoting resilience, healthcare workers can play a critical role in reducing the risk of suicide and improving the overall well-being of foster youth in the United States.

Role of Healthcare Workers in Supporting Foster Youth

Foster youth face unique challenges and vulnerabilities that can significantly impact their mental health and increase their risk of suicide. As healthcare workers, it is crucial for us to understand the role we play in supporting these young individuals within the foster care system. By providing them with comprehensive care, we can help alleviate their struggles and prevent tragic outcomes.

One of the key responsibilities of healthcare workers is to identify and address the mental health needs of foster youth. Research has consistently shown that this population is at a higher risk of developing mental health disorders such as depression, anxiety, and post-traumatic stress disorder (PTSD). By conducting thorough assessments and screenings, healthcare workers can identify these issues early on and initiate appropriate interventions.

By working closely with other professionals involved in the foster care system, healthcare workers can ensure that foster youth receive a holistic and coordinated approach to their care. Collaboration with social workers, psychologists, and other mental health providers is essential in developing individualized treatment plans that address the unique needs and challenges faced by foster youth.

In addition to providing mental health support, healthcare workers should also focus on the physical health of foster youth. Many of these individuals may have experienced neglect or abuse, leading to a higher prevalence of chronic health conditions. By addressing their physical health needs, healthcare workers can contribute to their overall well-being and reduce the burden of comorbidities on their mental health.

Education and training are vital components of supporting foster youth. Healthcare workers should be knowledgeable about the specific issues and risk factors that affect this population, including trauma, disrupted attachments, and loss. By understanding these factors, healthcare workers can provide culturally sensitive and trauma-informed care that promotes healing and resilience.

Furthermore, healthcare workers should advocate for policy changes and improvements within the foster care system. By actively participating in discussions and initiatives aimed at enhancing the support provided to foster youth, healthcare workers can contribute to systemic changes that address the root causes of their mental health struggles.

In conclusion, healthcare workers have a crucial role in supporting foster youth and preventing youth suicide. By providing comprehensive care, collaborating with other professionals, addressing both mental and physical health needs, and advocating for policy changes, healthcare workers can make a significant difference in the lives of these vulnerable individuals. Together, we can create a safer and more supportive environment for foster youth, reducing their risk of suicide and promoting their overall well-being.

Improving Mental Health Services for Foster Youth

Foster youth face unique challenges and are at a higher risk for mental health issues, including suicidal ideation and attempts. As healthcare workers, it is crucial to understand the specific needs of this vulnerable population and work towards improving mental health services for foster youth.

One of the key factors contributing to mental health disparities among foster youth is the instability they experience in their living situations. Moving from one foster home to another, often with limited support systems, can lead to feelings of abandonment, loss, and lack of stability. This constant upheaval can have detrimental effects on their mental well-being. Therefore, it is imperative to prioritize continuity of care for foster youth by ensuring that mental health professionals are accessible and available throughout their journey within the foster care system.

Another important aspect to consider is the trauma that many foster youth have endured before entering the system. Childhood abuse, neglect, and witnessing violence can have long-lasting psychological effects. Healthcare workers must be trained in trauma-informed care to approach these individuals with sensitivity and understanding. By creating a safe and supportive environment, healthcare professionals can establish trust and facilitate effective mental health interventions.

Additionally, collaboration and coordination among various stakeholders involved in the foster care system are crucial. Social workers, foster parents, teachers, and healthcare providers must work together to identify and address the mental health needs of foster youth. Regular communication and sharing of information can help identify warning signs and ensure appropriate interventions are in place.

Moreover, healthcare workers should advocate for policy changes that prioritize mental health services for foster youth. This includes adequate funding for mental health programs, training for foster parents and caregivers, and specialized support systems for those transitioning out of foster care. By actively engaging in advocacy efforts, healthcare workers can contribute to systemic changes that improve the overall mental well-being of foster youth.

In conclusion, improving mental health services for foster youth requires a multi-faceted approach. Healthcare workers must prioritize continuity of care, provide trauma-informed interventions, foster collaboration among stakeholders, and advocate for policy changes. By addressing the specific needs of foster youth, we can reduce mental health disparities and ultimately decrease the risk of youth suicide within this population.

Chapter 9: College Student Suicide in the United States

Stressors and Mental Health Challenges in College Settings

Introduction:

In today's fast-paced and competitive society, college can be a time of great excitement and personal growth for many young individuals. However, it is also a period that comes with its fair share of stressors and mental health challenges. This subchapter aims to shed light on the various stressors faced by college students and the resulting mental health issues. Understanding these challenges is crucial for healthcare workers who play a pivotal role in supporting and promoting the mental well-being of young adults.

Academic Pressure:

One of the primary stressors in college settings is academic pressure. Students often find themselves juggling multiple demanding courses, assignments, and exams. The fear of failure, competition, and the desire to excel academically can take a toll on their mental health. Healthcare workers must be aware of the signs of anxiety, depression, and burnout associated with academic stress and provide appropriate interventions.

Transition and Adjustment:

For many young adults, college marks a significant transition period, often involving leaving home, adapting to new surroundings, and building new social connections. This adjustment can be challenging and overwhelming, leading to feelings of loneliness, homesickness, and social isolation. Healthcare workers can assist by providing resources and support networks to help ease this transition and promote a sense of belonging.

Financial Burdens:

Financial strain is another significant stressor for college students, particularly for those from low-income backgrounds. The cost of tuition, textbooks, housing, and daily expenses can contribute to anxiety and distress. Healthcare workers can help by connecting students with financial aid resources, budgeting assistance, and counseling services to alleviate this burden.

Relationships and Social Pressures:

College is a time when young adults explore their identities and form new relationships. However, navigating romantic relationships, friendships, and social dynamics can be challenging and emotionally draining. Healthcare workers should be prepared to address issues related to unhealthy relationships, peer pressure, and the impact of social media on self-esteem and body image.

Balancing Responsibilities:

College students often find themselves juggling multiple responsibilities, such as academics, part-time jobs, extracurricular activities, and family obligations. The constant pressure to meet these demands can lead to feelings of overwhelm and exhaustion. Healthcare workers should emphasize the importance of self-care, time management, and stress management techniques.

Conclusion:

College settings can be breeding grounds for stressors and mental health challenges in young adults. Healthcare workers must be equipped with knowledge and resources to support college students in their mental well-being journey. By understanding the unique stressors faced by this population, healthcare workers can provide timely interventions, promote resilience, and ultimately help reduce the risk of youth suicide.

Campus-Based Suicide Prevention Initiatives

In recent years, the alarming rise in youth suicide rates in the United States has prompted healthcare workers to focus on implementing effective prevention strategies. One key aspect of these initiatives is the development of campus-based suicide prevention programs. These programs aim to create a supportive and inclusive environment for students, identify at-risk individuals, and provide timely interventions to prevent suicide.

One population that requires special attention is LGBTQ+ youth, as they face unique challenges that can contribute to their increased risk of suicide. Campus-based initiatives can play a crucial role in providing a safe and accepting space for LGBTQ+ students, offering support groups, counseling services, and educational programs to promote awareness and understanding.

Bullying has also been identified as a significant factor leading to youth suicide. Campus-based initiatives can work towards fostering a zero-tolerance policy for bullying, implementing anti-bullying programs, and offering counseling and support to victims. By creating a culture of respect and empathy, these initiatives aim to reduce the negative impact of bullying on students' mental health.

Minority youth, particularly those from marginalized communities, are disproportionately affected by suicide. Campus-based programs can address mental health disparities by providing culturally sensitive counseling services, outreach programs, and peer support groups tailored to the specific needs of minority students. By recognizing and addressing the unique challenges faced by these individuals, these initiatives can help reduce the incidence of suicide within these communities.

Rural areas and Native American communities often lack access to mental healthcare services, making them more vulnerable to suicide.

Campus-based initiatives can collaborate with local healthcare providers and community organizations to extend mental health support to these underserved populations. By leveraging their resources and expertise, these programs can bridge the gap and provide vital assistance to those in need.

College students, due to academic pressure and significant life transitions, are at increased risk of suicide. Campus-based initiatives can focus on raising awareness, providing mental health screenings, and offering counseling services specifically tailored to the needs of college students. By integrating suicide prevention efforts into the fabric of campus life, these initiatives can ensure that students receive the support they need during this critical period.

In the digital age, cyberbullying has emerged as a significant risk factor for youth suicide. Campus-based initiatives can collaborate with technology companies, educators, and parents to promote online safety, educate students about the harmful effects of cyberbullying, and provide resources for victims. By addressing this modern-day challenge, these programs can mitigate the negative effects of cyberbullying on mental health.

Lastly, for youth from military families and those in the foster care system, campus-based initiatives can provide tailored support services. By partnering with relevant organizations and agencies, these programs can ensure that these vulnerable populations receive the necessary mental health resources and interventions.

In conclusion, campus-based suicide prevention initiatives play a crucial role in addressing the complex factors contributing to youth suicide in the United States. By focusing on specific populations such as LGBTQ+ youth, victims of bullying, minority youth, rural communities, Native American communities, college students, victims of cyberbullying, and those from military families or in foster care, these initiatives can provide targeted support and interventions. By creating safe and inclusive environments, promoting awareness, and offering counseling services, campus-based programs can make a significant impact in reducing the incidence of youth suicide and promoting overall mental well-being.

Collaboration between Healthcare Workers and Universities

In the fight against youth suicide, collaboration between healthcare workers and universities is crucial. By working together, these two entities can pool their resources, expertise, and knowledge to develop effective prevention strategies and provide comprehensive care for at-risk youth. This subchapter explores the importance of collaboration between healthcare workers and universities in addressing the various facets of youth suicide in the United States.

Universities play a pivotal role in suicide prevention, particularly among college students. As educational institutions, they have direct access to this vulnerable population and can implement preventive measures, such as mental health screenings, counseling services, and educational programs. Healthcare workers, on the other hand, possess the clinical expertise to identify and treat mental health issues that may contribute to suicidal ideation. By collaborating, healthcare workers and universities can create a supportive environment that promotes mental well-being and early intervention.

Furthermore, collaboration is essential in addressing specific niches within youth suicide. For instance, LGBTQ+ youth face unique challenges that often contribute to higher rates of suicide. By partnering with universities known for their LGBTQ+ support programs, healthcare workers can leverage their resources to provide tailored care and support for this community. Similarly, collaboration between healthcare workers and universities can help tackle bullying-related youth suicide by implementing anti-bullying campaigns and fostering a culture of inclusivity.

Minority youth, rural communities, Native American populations, and those in the foster care system also require specialized attention when it comes to suicide prevention. Universities can conduct research to identify risk factors and cultural nuances, while healthcare workers can develop interventions that address the specific needs of these communities. By working together, they can bridge the gap in mental health disparities and provide equitable care for all youth.

Additionally, collaboration can address emerging challenges such as cyberbullying and military family youth suicide. Universities can contribute by conducting research on the impact of digital communication on mental health, while healthcare workers can develop protocols for identifying and treating cyberbullying victims. In the case of military families, universities can offer support programs for children and teens, while healthcare workers can provide mental health services that address the unique stressors faced by this population.

In conclusion, collaboration between healthcare workers and universities is essential in addressing youth suicide in its various forms. By combining their expertise, resources, and knowledge, these entities can develop comprehensive prevention strategies, provide tailored care, and bridge gaps in mental health disparities. Together, they can make a significant impact and save countless lives.

Chapter 10: Cyberbullying and Youth Suicide in the United States

Impact of Cyberbullying on Mental Health

Introduction:

In today's digital age, cyberbullying has emerged as a significant concern, particularly among the youth population. With the widespread use of technology and social media platforms, individuals are susceptible to online harassment, leading to severe consequences, including negative impacts on mental health. This subchapter aims to explore the profound impact of cyberbullying on mental health, presenting crucial insights for healthcare workers dealing with various niches of youth suicide in the United States.

1. Understanding Cyberbullying:

Cyberbullying refers to the deliberate and repetitive use of digital platforms to harm, intimidate, or harass individuals. It can manifest in various forms, including sending threatening messages, spreading rumors, sharing embarrassing images, or excluding someone from online groups. Healthcare workers must recognize the diverse ways in which cyberbullying can occur to effectively address its mental health implications.

2. Increased Risk of Depression and Anxiety:

Studies have consistently shown that victims of cyberbullying are at a higher risk of developing depression and anxiety disorders. Constant exposure to negative online interactions, humiliation, and social isolation can significantly impact a young person's mental well-being. Healthcare workers need to be aware of these risks and provide appropriate support and intervention to mitigate the adverse effects.

3. Suicidal Ideation and Self-Harm:

One of the most concerning consequences of cyberbullying is its association with suicidal ideation and self-harm among youth. The relentless nature of online harassment can lead vulnerable individuals to feel hopeless, trapped, and emotionally overwhelmed. Healthcare workers must be vigilant in identifying warning signs and providing timely intervention to prevent self-destructive behaviors.

4. Impact on Self-Esteem and Self-Image:

Cyberbullying often targets an individual's self-esteem and self-image, exacerbating feelings of inadequacy, shame, and worthlessness. Healthcare workers play a crucial role in helping young victims rebuild their self-confidence, fostering a positive sense of self, and promoting healthy coping mechanisms.

5. Long-Term Psychological Effects:

The impact of cyberbullying can extend beyond immediate mental health issues, leading to long-term psychological consequences. Victims may experience difficulties in forming healthy relationships, trust issues, and persistent anxiety even after the cyberbullying stops. Healthcare workers must provide ongoing support and therapy to address these long-lasting effects.

Conclusion:

Cyberbullying poses a severe threat to the mental health of young individuals across various niches of youth suicide in the United States. Healthcare workers need to be well-informed about the profound impact of cyberbullying on mental well-being to effectively identify and address the needs of their patients. By understanding the specific challenges faced by different populations, healthcare workers can play a critical role in preventing and mitigating the damaging effects of cyberbullying on youth mental health.

Preventive Measures and Online Safety Education

In today's digital age, online safety education is of paramount importance in preventing youth suicide. Healthcare workers play a crucial role in providing guidance and support to vulnerable individuals, particularly those belonging to high-risk groups such as LGBTQ+ youth, minority youth, rural youth, Native American youth, foster care system youth, college students, military families, and those affected by bullying or mental health disparities. This subchapter aims to equip healthcare workers with the necessary knowledge and tools to prevent youth suicide through effective preventive measures and online safety education.

One of the key preventive measures is early identification and intervention. Healthcare workers should be trained to recognize warning signs and risk factors associated with youth suicide, including social isolation, depression, anxiety, substance abuse, and previous suicide attempts. By identifying these signs early on, healthcare workers can provide timely support and intervention, connecting at-risk individuals with appropriate mental health resources.

Additionally, online safety education is crucial in today's interconnected world. Healthcare workers should educate youth about the potential dangers of cyberbullying, online harassment, and the impact of social media on mental health. They should provide guidance on responsible internet use, promoting positive online interactions, and fostering digital resilience.

Creating a supportive environment is another essential aspect of preventive measures. Healthcare workers should collaborate with schools, families, and communities to establish safe spaces where youth feel comfortable discussing their emotions and seeking help. By engaging in open dialogues, healthcare workers can raise awareness about the importance of mental health, reduce stigma, and encourage help-seeking behaviors.

Moreover, healthcare workers should advocate for accessible and culturally sensitive mental health services. They should be well-informed about the unique challenges faced by different high-risk groups, such as LGBTQ+ youth, Native American youth, and military families. By understanding their specific needs, healthcare workers can ensure that mental health services are tailored to address their concerns and promote positive mental well-being.

In conclusion, preventive measures and online safety education are vital in combating youth suicide. Healthcare workers have a crucial role in identifying at-risk individuals, providing timely interventions, and educating youth about online safety. By creating a supportive environment and advocating for accessible mental health services, healthcare workers can contribute significantly to reducing youth suicide rates among various high-risk groups in the United States.

Supporting Victims of Cyberbullying

In today's digital age, the prevalence of cyberbullying has become a significant concern, particularly when it comes to youth suicide in the United States. As healthcare workers, it is crucial that we are equipped with the knowledge and resources to support victims of cyberbullying effectively. This subchapter aims to provide a comprehensive understanding of cyberbullying and strategies for assisting victims, with a particular focus on the various niches related to youth suicide in the United States.

Cyberbullying refers to the act of using electronic communication platforms to harass, intimidate, or humiliate others. It can take many forms, including spreading rumors, sharing explicit content without consent, or constantly sending hurtful messages. LGBTQ+ youth, minority youth, and those in foster care or military families are particularly vulnerable to cyberbullying, which can exacerbate existing mental health disparities and increase the risk of suicide.

When dealing with victims of cyberbullying, healthcare workers should prioritize their safety and well-being. This involves creating a safe and nonjudgmental environment for victims to share their experiences. Active listening and empathy are critical in building trust and understanding the emotional impact of cyberbullying on victims. By validating their feelings and experiences, healthcare workers can help victims regain a sense of control and self-worth.

Additionally, healthcare workers should assess the severity of the cyberbullying and its impact on the victim's mental health. Collaborating with mental health professionals and counselors can provide victims with the necessary support and interventions. It may be beneficial to educate victims about coping mechanisms, such as stress reduction techniques, building resilience, and seeking social support from trusted individuals.

Furthermore, healthcare workers can play a vital role in raising awareness about cyberbullying and its consequences. By providing educational materials and conducting workshops, they can help communities understand the importance of fostering a safe and inclusive online environment. Collaborating with schools, parents, and online platforms can also contribute to the development of effective policies and preventive measures against cyberbullying.

In conclusion, supporting victims of cyberbullying requires a multifaceted approach that addresses the unique challenges faced by different populations, including LGBTQ+ youth, minority youth, and those in foster care or military families. By understanding the emotional impact of cyberbullying and providing appropriate support, healthcare workers can help reduce the risk of youth suicide related to cyberbullying.

Chapter 11: Mental Health Disparities and Youth Suicide in the United States

Disparities in Access to Mental Health Services

In recent years, there has been growing recognition of the alarming rates of youth suicide in the United States, with various subgroups facing unique challenges and vulnerabilities. Unfortunately, one significant barrier exacerbating this crisis is the disparities in access to mental health services. Healthcare workers must understand these disparities and work towards bridging the gap to ensure that all youth have equal opportunities to receive the care they need.

LGBTQ+ youth face disproportionate rates of suicide compared to their heterosexual peers. This can be attributed, in part, to the lack of culturally competent mental health services that understand and address the unique challenges faced by this community. Healthcare workers must not only create safe spaces for LGBTQ+ youth but also advocate for policies that promote inclusive care.

Bullying-related youth suicide is another concerning issue. Victims of bullying often suffer from mental health issues, yet they may not have access to the necessary support. Healthcare workers need to collaborate with schools and communities to implement effective bullying prevention programs and provide accessible mental health services for those affected.

Minority youth, including African American, Hispanic, and Asian American communities, also face disparities in access to mental health services. Language barriers, cultural stigma, and lack of culturally competent providers all contribute to limited access. Healthcare workers must actively engage with these communities, promote mental health awareness, and ensure that services are available in multiple languages.

Rural areas in the United States also experience significant disparities in mental health services. Limited healthcare facilities, transportation challenges, and a shortage of mental health professionals make it difficult for rural youth to access care. Telehealth initiatives and mobile mental health clinics can help bridge this gap and provide crucial services to these underserved populations.

Native American youth, foster care system youth, college students, and military families also face unique challenges that can contribute to mental health disparities and increased suicide rates. Healthcare workers must be aware of these specific needs and advocate for targeted resources and support systems to ensure these vulnerable populations receive the necessary care.

Furthermore, the impact of cyberbullying on youth suicide cannot be ignored. In the digital age, young people are exposed to online harassment and abuse, which can have severe consequences for their mental health. Healthcare workers must educate themselves about the effects of cyberbullying and work with schools, parents, and online platforms to address this issue effectively.

Addressing disparities in access to mental health services requires a multifaceted approach. Healthcare workers must advocate for policy changes, promote community awareness, collaborate with schools and organizations, and utilize innovative methods such as telehealth to reach underserved populations. By working together, we can ensure that all youth, regardless of their background, have equal opportunities to receive the mental health support they need and deserve.

Addressing Stigma and Barriers in Healthcare Systems

In the realm of youth suicide prevention, healthcare workers play a crucial role in identifying and addressing the numerous factors that contribute to this devastating issue. However, despite their best efforts, stigma and barriers within healthcare systems often hinder effective intervention and support. In this subchapter, we will explore the various forms of stigma and barriers that exist, specifically within the context of youth suicide in the United States. By understanding these challenges, healthcare workers can better equip themselves to provide the necessary care and support to at-risk individuals.

One significant area of concern is the stigma surrounding mental health and suicide. In many communities, mental health issues are still highly stigmatized, leading to shame, silence, and a reluctance to seek help. This stigma is even more pronounced within certain niches such as LGBTQ+ youth, minority groups, and Native American populations. Healthcare workers need to recognize and address these stigmas through education and community outreach programs. By fostering an environment of acceptance and understanding, we can encourage individuals to seek the help they desperately need.

Another barrier within healthcare systems is the lack of accessible mental health services, particularly in rural areas and within the foster care system. Limited resources, long wait times, and inadequate training for healthcare professionals often prevent timely intervention. It is imperative for healthcare workers to collaborate with policymakers and advocate for increased funding, improved infrastructure, and specialized training to effectively address these gaps in care.

In recent years, the rise of cyberbullying has become a significant concern, leading to an increased risk of youth suicide. Healthcare workers must recognize the unique challenges posed by this form of harassment and develop strategies to address it effectively. Collaboration with schools, parents, and social media platforms is crucial in implementing preventive measures and providing support to victims of cyberbullying.

Furthermore, mental health disparities among different populations, such as military families and college students, require targeted interventions. Understanding the unique stressors and challenges faced by these groups can help healthcare workers tailor their approach and provide targeted support.

In conclusion, addressing stigma and barriers in healthcare systems is essential for effective youth suicide prevention. Healthcare workers must work tirelessly to combat the stigma surrounding mental health, advocate for accessible services, and develop specialized interventions for at-risk populations. By doing so, we can create a healthcare system that is better equipped to provide the care and support necessary to prevent youth suicide and save lives.

Promoting Equity in Youth Suicide Prevention Efforts

In recent years, the issue of youth suicide has gained significant attention due to its devastating impact on individuals, families, and communities. While efforts to address this crisis have been made, it is crucial to recognize that not all youth face the same risk factors and challenges. To truly make a difference in preventing youth suicide, healthcare workers must promote equity in their prevention efforts.

One specific group that requires attention is LGBTQ+ youth. Studies have consistently shown that LGBTQ+ youth are at a higher risk of suicide compared to their heterosexual peers. Discrimination, bullying, and lack of acceptance contribute to the increased vulnerability of LGBTQ+ youth. Healthcare workers must actively work towards creating inclusive and supportive environments for these individuals, providing them with the resources and support they need to thrive.

Bullying is another significant risk factor for youth suicide. It is essential for healthcare workers to recognize the signs of bullying and intervene early to prevent tragic outcomes. By partnering with schools, parents, and community organizations, healthcare workers can implement comprehensive anti-bullying programs that promote empathy, respect, and kindness.

Minority youth, including African American, Hispanic, and Asian American youth, also face unique challenges that contribute to their increased risk of suicide. Healthcare workers must understand the cultural factors that impact mental health and suicide risk within these communities. By providing culturally sensitive care and addressing social determinants of health, healthcare workers can make a significant impact in reducing suicide rates among minority youth.

Rural communities in the United States often lack access to mental health services, making youth suicide prevention efforts particularly challenging. Healthcare workers must advocate for increased funding and resources to expand mental health services in rural areas. Telehealth initiatives and partnerships with community organizations can bridge the gap and ensure that youth in rural areas receive the support they need.

Native American youth, foster care system, college students, military families, and victims of cyberbullying are other niches that require specialized attention in youth suicide prevention efforts. Healthcare workers must collaborate with tribal communities, child welfare agencies, universities, military support organizations, and technology companies to develop tailored interventions and support systems.

Furthermore, mental health disparities and the intersectionality of various identities must be considered when designing and implementing suicide prevention efforts. Healthcare workers must address the root causes of these disparities, such as poverty, lack of access to healthcare, and systemic racism, to create a more equitable society where all youth have an equal chance at well-being.

In conclusion, promoting equity in youth suicide prevention efforts is crucial for healthcare workers. By addressing the unique challenges faced by LGBTQ+ youth, victims of bullying, minority youth, rural communities, Native American youth, youth in foster care, college students, victims of cyberbullying, individuals affected by mental health disparities, and military families, healthcare workers can make a significant impact in reducing youth suicide rates. It is only through these efforts that we can create a society where all youth have an equal opportunity for a healthy and fulfilling life.

Chapter 12: Military Family Youth Suicide in the United States

Unique Challenges Faced by Military Families

Military families often face unique challenges that can significantly impact the mental health and well-being of their children. Understanding these challenges is crucial for healthcare workers who aim to provide effective support and interventions for youth in military families.

One of the key challenges faced by military families is the frequent relocation and the resulting disruption of social connections. Military children often have to move to different states or even countries, which can lead to feelings of isolation, loss, and difficulty in making new friends. These frequent moves can contribute to a sense of instability and increase the risk of mental health issues and suicidal ideation among youth.

Another challenge is the prolonged separation from a parent who is deployed. Military deployments can last for months or even years, leaving children without the emotional and physical support of a parent. This separation can lead to increased stress, anxiety, and feelings of abandonment, increasing the vulnerability of youth to suicidal thoughts and behaviors.

Additionally, military families often experience high levels of stress due to the unique demands and uncertainties associated with military life. The constant worry about the safety of their deployed parent, financial strains, and the potential for sudden changes in family dynamics can create a stressful environment for children. These stressors can contribute to the development of mental health disorders, such as depression and anxiety, and increase the risk of suicide among youth in military families.

Furthermore, military families may face difficulties accessing mental healthcare services. In some cases, families may be located in remote areas with limited access to mental health professionals. Moreover, the stigma surrounding mental health within the military community may prevent families from seeking help when needed. These barriers to care can make it challenging for healthcare workers to provide timely and effective support to youth in military families.

In conclusion, healthcare workers need to be aware of the unique challenges faced by military families. By understanding the impact of frequent relocations, parental deployment, high levels of stress, and barriers to mental healthcare, healthcare workers can better support and advocate for the mental health needs of youth in military families. Through targeted interventions and accessible mental health services, healthcare workers can help reduce the risk of suicide among this vulnerable population.

Supporting Resilience and Mental Health in Military Youth

Introduction:

Military youth face unique challenges that can significantly impact their resilience and mental health. The constant relocation, parental deployment, and exposure to trauma can contribute to increased stress and vulnerability. As healthcare workers, it is crucial to understand the specific needs of these youth and provide effective support to promote their resilience and mental well-being.

Understanding the Impact:

Military youth often experience a range of emotions, including anxiety, loneliness, and fear, due to the unpredictable nature of military life. Multiple deployments and the potential loss of a parent can have a significant impact on their mental health. It is essential for healthcare workers to recognize these stressors and their potential consequences on youth suicide rates within military families.

Building Resilience:

Promoting resilience in military youth is crucial for their overall well-being. One effective approach is to provide access to support systems such as counseling services, peer support groups, and mental health resources. Encouraging healthy coping mechanisms, such as engaging in physical activity, creative outlets, and fostering positive relationships, can also contribute to building resilience.

Addressing Trauma:

Exposure to trauma is a common experience for military youth. Identifying and addressing trauma-related symptoms is essential to prevent the development of mental health disorders. Healthcare workers should be trained in trauma-informed care and evidence-based interventions to provide appropriate support to these youth.

Collaboration and Education:

Collaboration between healthcare workers, military personnel, and educators is crucial to provide comprehensive support to military youth. By sharing knowledge and resources, healthcare workers can ensure that these youth receive the necessary support both in and outside of the healthcare setting. Educating teachers and school staff about the unique needs of military youth can help create a supportive environment that promotes their mental health.

Promoting Cultural Competence:

Military families come from diverse backgrounds, including LGBTQ+ individuals, minority groups, and Native Americans. Healthcare workers should strive for cultural competence to understand the specific challenges faced by these groups. Tailoring interventions and support services to meet the unique needs of these populations can contribute to reducing youth suicide rates within their communities.

Conclusion:

Supporting resilience and mental health in military youth requires a comprehensive approach that addresses their unique challenges. By understanding the impact of military life, promoting resilience, addressing trauma, fostering collaboration, and promoting cultural competence, healthcare workers can play a vital role in reducing youth suicide rates within military families. It is our responsibility as healthcare workers to provide the necessary support and resources to ensure the well-being of these resilient and deserving youth.

Collaboration between Healthcare Workers and Military Services

In addressing the complex issue of youth suicide in the United States, it is essential for healthcare workers to collaborate closely with military services. The unique challenges faced by different populations, such as LGBTQ+ youth, minority youth, rural youth, Native American youth, foster care system-involved youth, college students, victims of cyberbullying, and those from military families, require a comprehensive approach that involves the expertise and resources of both healthcare professionals and military personnel.

The collaboration between healthcare workers and military services is particularly crucial when it comes to addressing mental health disparities among at-risk populations. Research has consistently shown that certain groups, such as LGBTQ+ youth, minority youth, and Native American youth, face higher rates of mental health issues and are more vulnerable to suicide. By working together, healthcare workers and military services can develop targeted interventions and support systems that address the unique needs of these populations, reducing the risk of youth suicide.

Furthermore, the collaboration between healthcare workers and military services is vital in understanding and addressing the specific factors that contribute to youth suicide within military families. The stressors associated with military life, such as frequent relocations, deployments, and the impact of parental mental health on children, can significantly increase the risk of suicide among military-connected youth. By joining forces, healthcare workers and military services can develop comprehensive prevention strategies, provide mental health support to military families, and ensure timely intervention for at-risk youth.

Additionally, the collaboration between healthcare workers and military services is essential in the prevention and management of bullying-related youth suicide. Bullying has emerged as a significant risk factor for suicide among young people, with both traditional and cyberbullying contributing to this devastating outcome. By working together, healthcare workers and military services can implement anti-bullying campaigns, educate communities about the detrimental effects of bullying, and establish effective reporting systems to protect vulnerable youth.

In conclusion, collaboration between healthcare workers and military services is vital in addressing the multifaceted issue of youth suicide in the United States. By pooling their expertise, resources, and experiences, healthcare professionals and military personnel can develop comprehensive prevention strategies, targeted interventions, and support systems that address the unique challenges faced by LGBTQ+ youth, minority youth, rural youth, Native American youth, foster care system-involved youth, college students, victims of cyberbullying, individuals affected by mental health disparities, and military families. Through this collaborative effort, we can make significant strides in reducing youth suicide rates and promote a healthier and more supportive environment for all young individuals in our society.

Chapter 13: Conclusion

Recap of Key Findings and Insights

In this subchapter, we will recap the key findings and insights from our comprehensive guide on understanding youth suicide. As healthcare workers, it is crucial to stay informed about the various aspects of youth suicide in the United States, and the niches of LGBTQ+ youth, bullying-related cases, minority groups, rural areas, Native American communities, foster care system, college students, cyberbullying, mental health disparities, and military families. By understanding the unique challenges faced by these groups, we can better address their needs and prevent tragic outcomes.

One of the key findings is the alarming prevalence of youth suicide in the United States. Despite ongoing efforts to raise awareness and provide resources, suicide remains the second leading cause of death among young people. This emphasizes the urgent need for healthcare workers to be proactive in identifying and addressing risk factors.

When it comes to LGBTQ+ youth suicide, our research reveals that they are particularly vulnerable due to the stigma, discrimination, and rejection they often face. Understanding the specific challenges they encounter can help healthcare workers create safe spaces and provide appropriate support.

Bullying has emerged as a significant risk factor for youth suicide. Our guide highlights the connection between bullying and suicidal ideation, emphasizing the importance of prevention and intervention programs in schools and communities.

Minority youth, including African American, Hispanic, and Asian American populations, are disproportionately affected by suicide.

Healthcare workers must consider cultural factors and develop culturally sensitive approaches to prevention and intervention.

Rural areas experience unique challenges in addressing youth suicide. Limited access to mental health resources, social isolation, and economic disparities contribute to higher rates of suicide. Healthcare workers must develop innovative strategies to reach and support youth in these underserved communities.

Native American youth face some of the highest rates of suicide in the United States. Understanding the historical and cultural factors that contribute to these rates is essential for healthcare workers to provide effective interventions and support.

The foster care system is another critical area where youth suicide rates are disproportionately high. Healthcare workers must collaborate with child welfare agencies to ensure proper mental health assessments, support, and resources for these vulnerable youth.

College students face significant stressors, including academic pressure, social challenges, and transitioning to adulthood. Healthcare workers should be aware of the warning signs and risk factors among this population and provide accessible mental health services on campuses.

The rise of cyberbullying has added another layer of complexity to the issue of youth suicide. Healthcare workers should collaborate with schools, parents, and online platforms to develop effective prevention and intervention strategies.

Mental health disparities among different racial and ethnic groups contribute to varying rates of youth suicide. Healthcare workers must advocate for equitable access to mental health resources and address systemic barriers.

Lastly, military families are confronted with unique stressors that can impact the mental health of young people. Healthcare workers should collaborate with military support services to provide comprehensive care and support for military youth.

By understanding these key findings and insights, healthcare workers can play a vital role in preventing youth suicide and promoting mental health among these diverse populations. It is essential to continue research, education, and collaboration to develop effective strategies and interventions that address the specific needs of each group. Together, we can make a significant impact and save lives.

Call to Action for Healthcare Workers

As healthcare workers, we have a critical role to play in addressing the alarming rates of youth suicide in the United States. The youth suicide crisis is a complex issue that affects various segments of our society, including LGBTQ+ youth, victims of bullying, minorities, those in rural areas, Native American communities, foster care system, college students, victims of cyberbullying, individuals facing mental health disparities, and military families. It is imperative that we take action to address these specific areas of concern and work towards preventing youth suicide across the nation.

First and foremost, we must prioritize education and awareness among healthcare workers. It is crucial that we stay informed about the unique challenges faced by different groups of at-risk youth. By understanding the specific risk factors, warning signs, and protective factors associated with LGBTQ+ youth, victims of bullying, minorities, rural communities, Native American communities, foster care system, college students, victims of cyberbullying, mental health disparities, and military families, we can better identify and intervene in potential suicide cases.

Additionally, collaboration and coordination among healthcare professionals, educators, social workers, and community leaders are essential. By establishing multidisciplinary teams, we can develop comprehensive prevention strategies tailored to the specific needs of each niche. This might involve creating safe spaces and support networks for LGBTQ+ youth, implementing effective anti-bullying programs in schools, providing culturally sensitive mental health services to minorities, improving access to mental health resources in rural areas, engaging Native American communities in suicide prevention efforts, addressing the unique challenges faced by youth in the foster care system, implementing mental health programs in colleges, combating cyberbullying through legislation and education, reducing mental health disparities through targeted interventions, and supporting military families through specialized programs.

Furthermore, healthcare workers should advocate for policy changes and allocate resources towards youth suicide prevention. By actively engaging in legislative efforts, we can push for comprehensive mental health reforms that prioritize early intervention, increase access to mental health services, and improve the quality of care. Additionally, we must advocate for increased funding for research into the underlying causes of youth suicide and the development of evidence-based prevention strategies.

In conclusion, healthcare workers have a crucial role to play in addressing the youth suicide crisis in the United States. By prioritizing education and awareness, fostering collaboration and coordination, and advocating for policy changes, we can make a significant impact in preventing youth suicide across various niches. Let us stand together and take action to save the lives of our nation's youth.

Future Directions in Youth Suicide Prevention Research and Practice

As healthcare workers, it is crucial for us to stay updated on the latest research and advancements in youth suicide prevention. By understanding the future directions in this field, we can better equip ourselves to address the specific needs and challenges faced by various populations of at-risk youth in the United States.

1. Youth Suicide in the United States: The future of youth suicide prevention research must focus on early identification and intervention strategies. This includes improved screening tools, risk assessment protocols, and the integration of mental health services within primary care settings.

2. LGBTQ+ Youth Suicide in the United States: Future research should prioritize understanding the unique experiences and risk factors faced by LGBTQ+ youth. It is essential to develop targeted interventions that address the specific mental health needs of this population, including fostering inclusive and supportive environments.

3. Bullying-Related Youth Suicide in the United States: Research and practice should emphasize the importance of comprehensive anti-bullying programs in schools, online platforms, and communities. Future directions should also explore the long-term effects of bullying and identify effective interventions for both victims and perpetrators.

4. Minority Youth Suicide in the United States: Culturally sensitive and inclusive approaches to suicide prevention are needed for minority youth populations. Future research should focus on developing culturally relevant interventions, addressing mental health disparities, and combating stigma within minority communities.

5. Rural Youth Suicide in the United States: Future directions should explore the unique challenges faced by rural youth, such as limited access to mental health services and isolation. It is crucial to develop innovative

approaches to reach these populations, including telehealth services and community-based prevention strategies.

6. Native American Youth Suicide in the United States: Culturally appropriate suicide prevention efforts should be a priority. Future research should emphasize community-based interventions, incorporating traditional healing practices, and strengthening connections to cultural identity and spirituality.

7. Foster Care System and Youth Suicide in the United States: Future directions should focus on improving the mental health support and services available to youth in the foster care system. Research should explore the impact of trauma-informed care and interventions that promote stability, resilience, and healthy coping strategies.

8. College Student Suicide in the United States: Future research should prioritize identifying the unique risk factors and developing targeted prevention strategies for college students. This includes increasing awareness of mental health resources on campuses, improving access to counseling services, and promoting mental health education.

9. Cyberbullying and Youth Suicide in the United States: Future directions should focus on developing effective prevention and intervention strategies for cyberbullying. This includes educating youth, parents, and educators about online safety, promoting responsible online behavior, and leveraging technology for positive mental health support.

10. Mental Health Disparities and Youth Suicide in the United States: Future research should examine the underlying factors contributing to mental health disparities among at-risk youth populations. It is crucial to develop interventions that address systemic inequalities, improve access to culturally competent care, and reduce stigma surrounding mental health.

11. Military Family Youth Suicide in the United States: Future directions should prioritize understanding the unique challenges faced by children and adolescents in military families. Research should focus on providing support and resources for military families, including mental health services, counseling, and community-based prevention programs.

In conclusion, the future directions in youth suicide prevention research and practice must encompass a comprehensive and targeted approach to address the diverse needs and challenges faced by at-risk youth populations in the United States. By actively engaging with these future directions, healthcare workers can contribute to the development of effective prevention strategies and interventions that save lives.